"CURRENTS AND COUNTER CURRENTS IN MEDICAL SCIENCE."

OLIVER WENDELL HOLMES, M. D.,

REVIEWED

IN AN

ADDRESS

DELIVERED BEFORE THE

Boston Academy of Homœopathic Medicine,

BY

ALBERT J. BELLOWS, M. D.,

Of Roxbury.

[SECOND EDITION.]

BOSTON:

PRINTED BY THE UNANIMOUS VOTE OF THE ASSOCIATION.

1860.

"CURRENTS AND COUNTER CURRENTS IN MEDICAL SCIENCE."

OLIVER WENDELL HOLMES, M. D.,

REVIEWED

IN AN

ADDRESS

DELIVERED BEFORE THE

Boston Academy of Homœopathic Medicine,

BY

ALBERT J. BELLOWS, M. D.,

Of Roxbury.

[SECOND EDITION.]

BOSTON:

PRINTED BY THE UNANIMOUS VOTE OF THE ASSOCIATION.

1860.

BOSTON:
John M. Hewes, Printer.
81 Cornhill.

"CURRENTS AND COUNTER CURRENTS IN MEDICAL SCIENCE."

In reviewing the Address of the learned Professor, whose motto I have borrowed, that which strikes the mind as most remarkable, is the fact, that after drifting in the "Currents and Counter Currents in Medical Science" for two thousand years, he finds himself just where he started,—trusting to nature and a good nurse.

Hippocrates, the acknowledged father of "Rational Practice," who wrote three hundred years before the Christian era, expressed so very exactly the "Professor's" sentiments, as to form, at least, a wonderful coincidence, the only discoverable difference being this; Hippocrates, "lest nature might be disturbed in her wholesome operation on the matter of disease," never, in any case, gave medicine till after the most active symptoms had subsided, while the Professor does make an exception in favor of three or four diseases, which the specifics are adapted to cure. The improvement in Rational Practice in two thousand years amounts then to simply this. A specific has been discovered for the itch, for syphilis and for intermittent fever, and possibly for some two or three other diseases; but they are not named by the Professor. Except the medicines adapted to cure these interesting diseases, so wonderfully favored by nature, the Professor firmly believes "that if the whole Materia Medica, *as now used*, could be sunk to the bottom of the sea, it would be all the better for mankind, and all the worse for the fishes." In justice, I ought to say, however, he does offer to "throw out" wine and opium, which Hippocrates undoubtedly used, and the anæsthetic vapors, which though not understood to cure disease, are undoubtedly a great blessing to mankind.

This, then, is the condition of Rational Medicine in the middle of the nineteenth century. There are known to be thousands of varieties of diseases, and thousands of varieties of medicines ; and a few of these diseases have medicines adapted to their cure ; but all the rest of the diseases are to be trusted to nature for cure, and all the rest of the medicines are to be thrown into the sea, as worse than useless. But have we not here a marvellous exception to the uniformity of nature's laws ?

We never find an eye, where there is not light to act upon it. And so uniform is this law, that fishes in the Mammoth Cave are made without eyes. We never find an ear, but where sound can put it in action. We never find a living thing, down to the invisible animalculæ, that has not its appropriate nourishment at hand. And is it not strange, that only a few of the thousands of diseases should have their appropriate remedies ? Shall we call that "Rational Medicine" which teaches that sulphur will cure the itch ; but denies that lime will cure a rash. Believes that mercury will cure syphilis ; but laughs at the idea of zinc as a remedy for herpes. Knows that Peruvian bark will cure intermittent fever ; but rejects the most positive testimony, that belladonna will cure scarlet fever ?

What can be the explanation of these inconsistencies ?

The Professor furnishes a good answer :—" It is so

hard to get any thing out of the dead hand of medical tradition."

Again, should that be called Medical Science, of which its own chosen Professor says, "The truth is, that medicine, professedly founded on observation, is as sensitive to outside influences, political, religious, philosophical, imaginative, as is the barometer to the changes of atmospheric density," and this he proves by eight or ten pages of historic facts, showing the innumerable opinions and theories, which have been set up, to be kicked over by the next man who should come along. Dr. Rush charging Hippocrates with killing millions, by letting nature loose upon sick people, and Sir John Forbes, Doctors Bigelow, Gould, Cotting, Hooker, and all other Hippocratic practitioners, holding Dr. Rush, and other heroic doctors, responsible for the lives of as many millions more. Not a substance under heaven, animal, vegetable, mineral or excrementitious, that has not been tried for medicine, and not one that has not, in its turn, been condemned as injurious or useless, and this while all other branches of science have been steadily progressing,—Astronomy, chemistry, geology, constantly adding new principles and new facts, having no "counter currents," and never subject "to outside influences, political, religious or imaginative."

But geology never did much while its "dead hand" held on to misinterpreted theology. Chemistry made no advances, while it amused itself by chasing the phantoms of alchemy. Astronomy stood still till Galileo's telescope revealed the simple law which governs it. And Medical Science is drifted every where by "currents and counter currents," till it recognises the simple law of nature, which God, in infinite mercy, has given to guide it. "*Similia similibus curantur.*" But wherever this law is recognized, the Science of Medicine has progressed as steadily as any other science.

Look at the Materia Medica of the two systems, as they have been developed by the last fifty years of time. Hundreds of articles have been tested by allopathic physicians on the sick, and thousands of patients have been killed in the experiments, as the doctors themselves acknowledge, and not a half dozen of all the medicines have continued in general use for any consecutive ten years of practice; while every article of well proved homeopathic medicine which was used fifty years ago is used now by every homeopathic physician. And of the hundreds of articles which have since been proved, by experiment, (not on the sick, but on ourselves, thus avoiding the sacrifices consequent on allopathic experiments,) not one that has been fairly proved to be useful is ever afterwards condemned or abandoned.

Chemical laws are no more certain in their operation, than is the homeopathic law, and this I assert after twenty consecutive years of practice in experimental chemistry. I am no more sure that an appropriate quantity of acid will neutralize a given quantity of alkali, than I am sure that a medicine which in large doses will produce a headache, will in small doses cure a similar headache. Chemistry, therefore, to my mind, is no more entitled to be ranked as a science, than is homeopathy.

Again, since the promulgation of the homeopathic law, thousands of educated men have tested it in practice; but not one of them ever found a fact or an argument to disprove it; or, after the trial of a single year, ever disbelieved it. The idea of turning back a true disciple of

Hahnemann to a belief in allopathy, or Rational Medicine, is as preposterous as the idea of turning a disciple of Galileo to a belief in the old Ptolemaic system of astronomy. Some sage cotemporary might say to Galileo, I don't believe in your philosophy, for the world could not turn round without spilling the water from my well; but Galileo would reply, as he did, "Nevertheless, the world does turn round, and I can prove it." So some equally sage Professor may say, I don't believe in homeopathy, for I have never seen much effect on the waters of Lake Superior by a drowned louse; nevertheless, the law, "*Similia similibus curantur*," is true, and we can prove it; and this is all we claim for homeopathy. Our Professor says Hahnemann believed in infinitesimal doses, and in psora as the origin of many chronic diseases; and "does not Hahnemann himself represent homeopathy as it now exists?" "He, certainly ought to be its best representative," &c. Admit that Hahnemann, in his dotage, did believe and publish some foolish things, is homeopathy responsible for them, even while they were never adopted as the homeopathic creed? then is Rational Medicine responsible for every foolish thing its Professors believe and publish. Let us try on a case, and see how it fits. I cannot believe, with the rationalist, that typhoid fever resides on the mucous membrane of the tongue, and can be scraped off with a hoe. And does any rational practitioner say, neither do I believe such nonsense; but "does not" your own Professor of your own favorite school, "represent" Rational Medicine "as it now exists?" "He certainly ought to be its best representative." And does he not, in this very Address, recommend a hoe as a very economical remedy,*

* Address by O. W. Holmes, M. D. Page 23.

"better than many a prescription with a split-footed ℞ before it?" And does he not enforce his recommendation by a very interesting scrap of Colonial history, the pith of which is, that Winslow scraped the tongue of Massasoit, then like to die of typhoid fever, and thus saved his life, and with it the Colony? Here is proof that the Professor believes that typhoid fever resides on the tongue; for how else could it be scraped off. And thus we establish the very important discovery in Rational Medicine,—typhoid fever is a disease of the tongue, and a hoe will cure it. Now, ridiculous as is this representation of Rational Medicine, it is less a caricature than any published representation of homeopathic doctrines, which I can find from the pen of any allopathic practitioner within the last twenty years. See the Professor's representation of us in this very Address.

After charging us with "outraging human nature with infusions of *pediculus capitis*; that is, of course, as we understand their dilutions, the names of these things; for if a fine-tooth-comb insect were drowned in Lake Superior, we cannot agree with them in thinking that every drop of its waters would be impregnated with all the pedicular virtues they so highly value." He says, "They know what they are doing,—they are appealing to the detestable old superstitious presumption in favor of whatever is nauseous and noxious as being good for the sick." Here are three distinct misrepresentations of us in one sentence:—

1st. We are represented as "outraging human nature" and appealing to the vulgar and "superstitious presumption in favor of whatever is nauseous," and this under a Latin name, and "in infinitesimal sugar globules," while, in the very preceding paragraph, he has been referring to the allopathic use of medicines, "transcendently unmentionable," and of "unlovely secretions" which were used undiluted.

2d. We are represented as believing that a louse, drowned in any part of Lake Superior, would impregnate its waters a hundred miles off, against all "currents and counter currents," a belief which Hahnemann, in his last days of dotage, of course, never thought of.

3d. We are represented as highly valuing the virtues of the "*pediculus capitis*," when it cannot be found in any list of homeopathic remedies, and I venture the assertion, was never used by a homeopathic physician in any dilution. As a homeopathic remedy, it seems to have come from the *head* of his friend, Dr. Martin, who charges us with hooking it from the allopathic Materia Medica, with fifty other articles, some of which are among our most valuable remedies; this one, however, he acknowledges he cannot find in our list of remedies, or any where else; but he *understands* "it enjoys a distinguished place in homeopathic pharmacy."†

This address, by the way, affords another illustration of the usual method of attack on homeopathy, by misrepresentation and ridicule, rather than by facts or arguments. The main purpose seems to be to show that homeopathy did not originate with Hahnemann. And this he attempts to do by hunting up all the medicines from the animal, vegetable or mineral kingdoms, used by Hahnemann, and then going back hundreds of years to see how many of the same medicines had been used before Hahnemann was born. But as he finds among allo-

---

† See Address of Henry A. Martin, M. D., of Roxbury, before the Norfolk County Medical Society. Page 26.

pathic medicines *every thing under heaven*, he has left poor Hahnemann no other resources but the allopathic Materia Medica, and what does he prove by that process ?

But what seems most to amuse the doctor, is, that he finds Hahnemann guilty of hooking from their Materia Medica, inert substances, as gold, antimony, tin, silicea, &c., and pretending to perform wonderful cures with them, after trituration with sugar ; but does he forget that lead and mercury are equally inert substances ? What is his blue pill, which has cured so many and killed so many patients, but crude mercury, (of which a pound could be taken with impunity,) and conserve of roses perseveringly triturated together ? Apropos to our triturations, which are sources of such infinite amusement, let us remind him of the well known fact, that allopathic doctors attribute the power of the blue pill to such a minute division of the mercurial particles, as to adapt them to the capacity of the absorbent vessels. Whether their theory is right or not, every homeopathic physician knows that gold, and charcoal, and silicea, and many other inert substances, are made valuable medicines by a similar process, using only sugar instead of conserve of roses.

The address closes with deep regrets that he had so exhausted the time in these, to him, very interesting researches, that he could not, as he intended, bring out his plan for punishing such incorrigible quacks ; but whether it was his design to punish them for hooking his "*pediculus capitis*," or for copying his placebo practice, he does not inform us. One or the other it must be, for neither he nor his cotemporaries charge us with any worse sins.

Neither does the original exponent of Rational Medicine in New England, ever refer to homeopathy, to my knowledge, without misrepresenting it. In his last work on Rational Medicine, he even charges us with being faithless to our principles.* He says, "There is great reason to believe that homeopathic faith is not always kept up to its original purity by its professors ; traces of the occasional use of very heroic medicines are often detected," &c.

Will the doctor be kind enough to refer to any article of homeopathic faith that specifies the size or strength of the dose at all ; the only rule is to give enough to produce the effect desired. And now that the doctor is up, let me relieve his mind on another point. He says, on the same page, "The man must be somewhat of a stoic, who can look upon a case of severe colic, and quiet his conscience with administering inappreciable globules instead of remedies." Now let me tell my kind-hearted old friend and teacher, what I know to be true, after repeated experiments, both in accordance with the Rules of Bigelow's Sequel and those of homeopathy, that a homeopathic remedy will relieve the severest colic in one quarter of the time of his own most heroic opiate ; often before it could be obtained from the nearest druggist. Opium is the slow coach, for which we are not willing to wait.

But is not the dose which homeopathic practitioners generally give, so ridiculously small as to justify the definition given to our system by expositors of Rational Medicine "as a specious mode of doing nothing ?" To one accustomed to the use of ipecac, for example, in twenty grain doses, it may seem impossible that the one thousandth part of a grain of the same article can produce any effect ; but how is it known that twenty grains

---

* Expositions of Rational Medicine. By Jacob Bigelow, M. D.

will produce an emetic effect, but by experiment; and experiment as clearly shows that the one thousandth part of a grain of ipecac will as surely stop vomiting, when produced by some other cause. And how can the Professor know, or any one else, whether the ten thousandth part of a grain might not also produce an effect? Theoretically, who shall decide whether the crude article, third, or thirtieth dilution, is best adapted to the capacity and size of the invisible capillaries, in which it must circulate and on which it must act; or whether one dilution may not be best adapted to diseases of one tissue, and another to diseases of a different tissue. We can easily ridicule the high dilutions, but who shall settle that old question of divisibility, so as to tell us in which dilution, from the third to thirtieth, the original material has ceased to exist, or existing, is too fine to be adapted to the infinitesimal vessels of which the tissues are composed. Take, for example, sulphate of copper, one grain of which can be seen intermingled with every drop of five gallons of water, which may be equal to the fifth dilution. Does it cease to exist in the sixth dilution, because it cannot be seen? And who knows the nature of the specific action of medicines, whether it may not be increased by the increase of surface produced by each dilution, just as the power of electricity may be increased by extending the surface. The action of medicine is a mystery always, and is it profitable to ridicule that of which we know nothing?

And how do the specifics act in the cure of disease? All classes of practitioners have seen the hundredth part of a grain of corrosive sublimate, given in repeated doses, gradually change a diseased action to a healthy action. Call this an alterative, or call it a homeopathic action.—

What is it ? In Bigelow's Sequel you are told, " Alteraative is a name applied to substances which are found to produce a change in the system favorable to recovery from disease." And he gives, as examples, arsenic, sulphur, mercury. The same articles, it will be remembered, which are mentioned by our Professor as the specifics, and these articles are found to produce their effect in very small doses. Here is homeopathy on a small scale. Two or three hundred articles beside those mentioned by the Professor and the Doctor, are also known to homeopathic practitioners to " produce a change in the system favorable to recovery from disease," and their number is constantly increasing, and the fair inference is, that all other medical substances are intended to act in the same way on their own appropriate diseases. But Rational practitioners and Rational professors can see no common sense in homeopathy. Will the Professor's six methods of " misapplying the evidence of nature," give us a clue to the reason of this anomaly. Let us see :—

First. " There is the natural incapacity for sound observation." " We see this in many persons who know a *good deal about books*, but who are not sharp-sighted enough to buy a horse or deal with human diseases." A truth that cannot be better illustrated than by reference to the treatment of typhoid fever with a hoe.

Secondly. " There is, in some persons, a singular inability to weigh the value of testimony, of which, I think, from a pretty careful examination of his books, Hahnemann affords the best specimen outside of the walls of bedlam." That Hahnemann is the best specimen this side of bedlam, we certainly cannot agree, for we have seen a Professor who believes, from mere tradition, that a hoe will cure typhoid fever ; but ridicules the testimony of hundreds of educated physicians, that belladonna will cure a sore throat, and aconite a fever.

Thirdly. "We are led into inveterate logical errors, by counting only favorable cases." And here the Professor supplies an illustration. If an Indian chief gets well of typhoid fever after hoeing out his mouth, his case is reported; but nothing is said of the other poor Indians who died in spite of the scraping.

Fourthly. "The *post hoc ergo propter hoc* error." "That is, He got well after taking medicine, therefore, in consequence of taking it." Let us look again to the same source for illustration. Massasoit got well after scraping his tongue, therefore, the hoe saved his life, "and saved the Colony, and thus rendered Massachusetts and the Massachusetts Medical Society a possibility." "*Post hoc ergo propter hoc.*"

Lastly. "A reason for the golden tooth,"—"that is, assuming a falsehood for a fact, and giving reasons for it." This the Professor illustrates by the "homeopathic Materia Medica." But the homeopathic Materia Medica is founded on proof, and nothing but proof admits a single article. But what well attested fact is his own hoe theory founded on? Indeed, every practical physician knows the statement to be untrue, "that the condition of the tongue does not in the least imply that of the stomach." Let the Professor practice physic for a single year, and he will be as anxious to buy up his address of 1860, as he now is to purchase that of 1842.*

Nor is that other dogma of "Rational Medicine,"

---

* Wanting a copy of Homeopathy and its Kindred Delusions, to preserve as a curiosity, a friend found with an antiquarian a single copy; but it could be had for no less than one dollar; for he said the author would pay that for all he could get.

which is brought out by Dr. Bigelow, distinctly stated by Dr. Gould, commented on and enforced by Dr. Cotting, and ludicrously re-stated by our Professor, less repugnant to nature's common laws. "Drugs, in themselves considered, may always be regarded as evils." Four or five drugs are known to rational practitioners under the name of alteratives, or specifics, "to produce a secret change in the system favorable to recovery from disease," and this in doses so small as to be tasteless, and to produce no perceptible evils; and hundreds are equally well known to us, to produce similar effects under the name of "homeopathic remedies." And is it reasonable to suppose that other drugs are intended by Nature to effect a cure only by producing such serious evils as to make it a question, whether the effects of the medicine, or the effects of the disease, are most to be feared? Is it not more "rational" to suppose that drugs, like every other blessing from God, are intended for good, and for good only? and that the wrong application of them produces the evils which are known to result from them? For illustration, in testing my old allopathic drugs in homeopathic practice,—and this is the best use to which I can apply my allopathic knowledge,—I find constant corroborations of this belief.

In using rhubarb or calomel, for example, as I often did in operative doses, for the cure of diarrhœa; the patient was reduced and his digestive functions were deranged, but the disease was cured, and until I learned the truth, I was reconciled to the evils on account of the benefits of the medicine; but I now find rhubarb or calomel much more useful in the same disease in doses too small to reduce the patient or derange his digestive functions; and the inference to my mind is fair, that in allopathic doses, the cure was effected in spite of the active operation, and not on account of it. I have tested many medicines in the same way, with this uniform result,—where large doses of medicine will cure a disease, with accompanying evils, small doses will accomplish the same end without such evils.

And yet so universal is the opinion, that medicine can do no good except in a form in which it is capable of doing harm, that we meet this argument against homeopathic medicine every where. "I knew of a child that swallowed a whole bottleful, and it did him no harm," and this is supposed to settle all controversy on this subject. The sick cat eats with apparent relish the few leaves of the simple medicine which nature furnishes it, and gets well without accompanying evils ; but the poor sick child must swallow drugs which it shudders to think of, and which disturb every function for days and weeks, and sometimes for life ; because nature furnishes medicine for man in a crude, unpalatable condition. Why not, for the same reason, take our food as nature furnishes it, in a crude, unpalatable condition ? We use our reason in preparing food which is adapted to supply the wants of our nature ; and when we have succeeded, we are rewarded by the consciousness of its adaptation. So God evidently intended we should use our reason in adapting medicines to the cure of the diseases for which they were intended, and when we succeed, we are also rewarded with the evidence of their adaptation. Every homeopathist has been gratified with this evidence, sometimes in five minutes after the medicine is taken, and the more violent the disease, the more frequent is relief almost immediate. If, instead of relief, we get evils, we may be sure we have mistaken the appropriate remedy, or have given it in an improper condition, just as we are always sure we have taken improper food, or have taken it in an improper condition, when, instead of gratified appetite, we have loathing and disturbance from it.

Is it reasonable, that while our Heavenly Father gives us a relish for every thing that is good for us in health, He should give us a disgust for any thing necessary for us in sickness ? Our reason, therefore, as well as our humanity and our experience, demand that every thing offensive, in diet, regimen or medicine, should be excluded from the sick chamber.

But suppose our system is " a specious mode of doing nothing," and our " Materia Medica sugar of milk and a nomenclature." Are we sinners above all others ? By their own showing we carry out the plan of Hippocrates, and Bigelow, and Cotting, and the Professor himself; for we certainly give nature a fair chance, and our " rules of diet and nursing are excellent," Miss Nightingale being judge (and her authority, will, of course, be accepted by the Professor, who places her name next to that of Hippocrates). What, then, is the offence for which we are treated with such contempt by our allopathic brethren ? Why, we give sugar of milk, and make our patients think we are doing something for them. That we use the slightest deception, is not true ; but, if it were, are we the only practitioners who deceive patients with " sugar of milk and a nomenclature ?"

Look at the piles of prescriptions, put up every day by every apothecary in Boston, and remember, that according to the Professor, you are at the American head-quarters of the " nature-trusting " practice. How many of them contain any thing more important than sugar of milk, with, perhaps, a little coloring matter ? And remember that every prescription costs the patient from twenty-five to fifty cents, while our medicine costs the patient nothing, and then ask "Dr. Howe's least promising pupil," whether the homeopathic or the rational practitioner is most amenable to the charge of deceiving with placebo medicines. And that is all the charge that our worst enemies bring against us. By this comparison, it will be seen, I have presented the worst view of homeopathy, and the best view of allopathy.

For while it is evident, as I have shown, that one class of practitioners is every day practising deception, by writing placebo prescriptions, to be paid for, in which they have not themselves the slightest confidence, (the only object being to please the patient, while nature cures the disease); another class is doing infinitely worse, writing for medicines, to be paid for, which actually do very great harm. That too much medicine is given, the Professor proves, by reference to the undisputed fact, that doctors and their families take little or no medicine, and, for the inference from this fact, he appeals to "the least promising of Doctor Howe's pupils." And here, by the way, I wish to present to the same sapient umpire, a counter statement, equally true. Homeopathic physicians and their families do take their own medicine, and in precisely the same doses and dilutions as their other patients take them. Apropos to the charge of deception, I will state a bit of experience. For fifteen years up to 1845, I practised medicine in the confidence of the Massachusetts Medical Society; and, like most of my fellows, I gradually lost confidence in medicine, till my practice was as harmless as the most perfect "nature-trusting" practitioner of Boston or vicinity; but my conscience gave me so much trouble, while practising the deception, absolutely necessary in order to retain my patients till nature cured the disease, that I wrote my last placebo prescription in 1845, resolving that come what would, I would live in peace with conscience. Having thus cast off the fear of the Medical Society, I was enabled to look at facts all about me, showing the truth and the success of homeopathy, and the result was an honest adoption of its principles and its practice.

And now having no occasion for deception, in order to retain my patients, and giving no medicine but with the honest purpose and expectation of curing disease, or at least of assisting nature in doing so, and receiving almost daily acknowledgments of cure, where nature and heroïc remedies have all failed, I enjoy the practice of medicine as I did not think it possible, while in Allopathic or Rational Practice. True, it is not pleasant to see such epithets as "Arrant Quackery," "Infinitesimal Humbug," "Solemn Farce," "Pretended Science," &c., applied to that system, which, next to the *Christian religion*, we esteem the best gift of God to man ; but when we see, as in the Professor's last address, these opprobrious terms applied to us in six different places, without one fact or argument to show their application, we believe, as every body else believes, that facts and arguments would not be withheld, but for the want of them. And when these very men, who send every day prescriptions, to be paid for, which they know to be worthless, refuse to consult with us in cases of surgery, or obstetrics, where we should not differ in practice, making no other charge against us than that we give "sugar of milk ;" we can heartily join, with our intelligent neighbors, in the laugh at their ridiculous position, especially as they who *win* are always allowed to laugh.

A case of the latter kind occurred recently in my own practice, sufficiently instructive, not to say amusing, to warrant a brief narration. A lady in one of our best families, a favorite in a large circle of friends, was in a condition almost desperate ; and wanting advice and assistance, I recommended a friend of great experience in such cases ; but in the consternation of the neighborhood, and in the absence of the husband, each kind-hearted neighbor proposed sending for *her* doctor, as all would then be safe. One ran for an old allopathic friend of the family ; but he absolutely refused to go to the house, even to save the life of a daughter of an old friend. Another was hastily sent for, who happened to be my junior in the Harvard School, and my junior in the Medical Society, Dean of the Faculty, Professor of Obstetrics, &c., &c. He *would go*, as an act of humanity, but with the distinct understanding that he did not consult with a homeopathic physician. He did go, and walking, with solemn tread, into the chamber, he "whipped the devil around the stump," by looking straight at the bed-post, at which I was standing, and consulting *that* and giving to *that* his advice ; thus ingeniously evading the medical law, but, apparently, not quite satisfying his own conscience ; for he went out of the house as if the very —— Medical Society was at his heels ; kindly hinting that he should be willing to call again, and do what could be done for the suffering patient, provided the homeopathic doctor could be disposed of. The father, himself not a believer in homeopathy, indignant at the "solemn farce," said to me, "I can stand no more of this nonsense ; do what you think best, get what assistance you choose, and I will take the responsibility;" shrewdly inquiring if these doctors had not lost patients by homeopathy. And his intimation that the Medical Society was not fully responsible for all he had seen and heard, was corroborated by the fact, that another friend of the family, a physician of high standing, had heard of no law against consulting with an educated physician, if he did give sugar pills instead of placebo prescriptions. The result was, a free and gentlemanly attendance and assistance, till, by the blessing of God on a course of treatment, quite different from that recommended through the bed-post, our patient recovered.

Here let us leave "The Currents and Counter Currents in Medical Science," and borrowing the motto of another celebrated author and poet, close by recounting, very briefly, "The Happy Success of the Valiant Knight, and his Dreadful and Inconceivable Adventures; with other Incidents worthy to be Recorded by the most able Historian."

The crusade against homeopathy in New England was commenced in 1841, and was announced in these words, "I shall treat it, not by ridicule, but by argument;" "with a firm belief that its pretensions and assertions cannot stand before a single hour of calm investigation.*"

The address is commenced with the acknowledgment that "The one great doctrine which constitutes the basis of homeopathy, as a system, is expressed by the Latin aphorism, '*similia similibus curantur*.'" And yet, without bringing a single argument against this one great doctrine, he devotes the rest of his lecture to a mere

---

* Homeopathy and its Kindred Delusions. Page 27.

effigy, which he makes up of rags and shreds from the mind of Hahnemann in his dotage, which he labels homeopathy ; but which is as unlike homeopathy as Don Quixote's windmills were unlike the giants, for which he mistook them.

In a western village, where Republicanism is carrying all before it, the papers say some sapient politicians adopted a new and safe way of combating it. They obtained some old clothes, stuffed them with straw, and labelling their effigy 'Old Abe,' danced around it like the Professor's typhoid Indians, "making such a hellish noise as they probably thought would scare away the devil of"* Republicanism. They finally pelted it with stones, and, demolishing it, seemed to think they had put an end to Republicanism. So our hero, having in less than an hour demolished his own effigy of Hahnemann, thought he had kept his engagement, and demolished homeopathy past resuscitation ; for he gravely proceeded to post-mortem arrangements. This part of the service is sufficiently amusing to warrant a copy of the programme verbatim, with a few running commentaries.

The Professor says, "It only remains to throw out a few conjectures as to *the particular manner* in which it is to break up and disappear."

"1st. The confidence of the few believers in this delusion will never survive the loss of friends, who may die of any acute disease, under a treatment such as that prescribed by homeopathy. It is doubtful how far cases of this kind will be trusted to its mercies ; but wherever it acquires any considerable foothold, such cases must

---

* Address of O. W. Holmes, M. D., May 30, 1860. Page 23.

come, and, with them, the ruin of those who practice it, should any highly valuable life be thus sacrificed."

Well, nineteen years have passed since this terrible doom was assigned us, and who has been ruined ? Who has even been alarmed ?

"2d. After its novelty has worn out, the ardent and capricious individuals, who constitute the most prominent class of its patrons, will return to visible doses, were it only for the sake of a change."

As a commentary on this prophecy, I simply challenge contradiction to the following statement:—For every family that gives up homeopathy for allopathy, twenty give up allopathy for homeopathy.

"3d. The semi-homeopathic practitioner will gradually withdraw from the *rotten half* of his business, and try to make the public forget his connection with it."

This prophecy has proved literally true ; but not exactly in the manner intended by the prophet. Every man of us, who began practising both ways, (and nine-tenths of us began that way,) finding by experience that homeopathic practice is the most reliable, safe and expeditious mode of curing disease, have gradually withdrawn from allopathy, till, after a very few years, we give up "*the rotten half*" altogether ;—to this there is not a known exception. And one benevolent gentleman, who, when the prophecy was published, was practising both ways, now is, and for years has been, practising homeopathy only, and from mere motives of benevolence, taking fees from no one.

"4th. The ultra homeopathist will either recant and try to rejoin the medical profession ; or he will embrace some newer, and, if possible, equally extravagant doctrine ; or he will stick to his colors and go down with his sinking doctrine. *Very few will pursue the course last mentioned.*"

When this prediction was published, there were probably in Massachusetts, seven or eight educated homeopathic physicians, now there are, according to allopathic testimony, over two hundred ; then there were in the United States probably one hundred, now probably at least three thousand ; then the prophet had just reported homeopathy in Paris to be in a " condition sufficiently miserable," to use his own words, and going down, as it was, also, according to the same authority, in England and Germany. Now, I am informed by an intelligent gentleman, who has travelled in all the countries mentioned, that there are in Paris one hundred educated homeopathic practitioners, and in every place where homeopathy has obtained a foothold, it has steadily progressed. Not a man of all this army of homeopathic physicians has ever been known to recant, and not one has embraced any newer doctrine, extravagant or otherwise, except as an adjuvant to homeopathy.

" Lastly. Not many years can pass away before the same curiosity, excited by one of Perkins's tractors, will be awakened at the sight of one of the " infinitesimal globules." " If it should claim a longer existence, it can only be by falling into the hands of the sordid wretches, who wring their bread from the cold grasp of disease and death, in the hovels of ignorant poverty."

Twenty years ago, pure globules, prepared for medication, were imported by the pound ; now they are made in this country, and sold by the hundred, if not by the ton. And is it from sordid wretches, of ignorant poverty, such as passed before the seer's vision, that the fifteen thousand dollars, for Dispensary purposes, have recently come, when we only asked for five thousand? And are our patients all of that wretched class? Why, it is only a few weeks since some of us heard this same seer publicly charging the Governor of our Commonwealth with being guilty of placing his valuable life in the hands of homeopathy.

Thus ends the story of the first valiant attack in which homeopathy is not only ignominiously killed, but shockingly dismembered; but Banquo's ghost never was half so troublesome to poor Macbeth, as has since been the ghost of Hahnemann to our Professor. It not only *gets into his chair*, at public dinners, but into his *medical chair*, and at his "Breakfast Table;"—wherever he is, up comes this phantom to plague him, till we can say, as the Salem Register says of the phantom of old John Brown and the Editor of the Boston Courier. We are afraid that poor old Hahnemann, "who is dead and gone, will yet be the death of him." Well, homeopathy being thus disposed of, "nothing remains" but a very brief notice of some valiant attacks on the advocates of it.

We have already referred to the plan of extermination, by refusing to consult with us; but, that failing, we have been not a little amused at another device still more ridiculous. This plan was first made public in 1859, when, after a year of preparation, the Berkshire Professor brought out his big gun.*

After acknowledging the impotence of other persecutions, he says, "I would expel them as quacks," (the cream of this joke is, very few of us attend their meetings or take an interest in their proceedings. They can expel us from the privilege of paying three dollars a

---

* Address by Dr. Timothy Child of Pittsfield, May 20, 1859.

year, for a dinner which we never eat, that is all.) But what is a quack? An ignorant pretender? That won't do, for some of them graduated at our college, and none of them pretend to knowledge, which they are not willing to communicate to the whole world. Well, we must get up a definition that will hit them. "The essence of quackery is, ignoring the wisdom and guidance of the past, and assuming and advertising to be possessed of a skill beyond our contemporaries." But don't the doctor see who stands in the range of this shot. Our Professor so far "ignores the wisdom and guidance of the past," as to propose to throw into the sea almost the entire Materia Medica, which has been accumulating for over two thousand years. And he assumes and advertises a skill in the cure of typhoid fever, that not one of his contemporaries ever dreamed of. And Louis, a name which the doctor can't mention but with profound respect, is also a consummate quack, for he ignores all wisdom, past and present, and sets up a system of his own; and Hunter, Harvey, Newton, Galileo, and old Hippocrates himself, are all quacks, and, according to this definition, *worse* quacks than Hahnemann or any of his disciples.

> "His gun, well aimed at duck or plover,
> Bears wide and knocks its owner over."

Well, the Society meets and passes a vote of thanks to Dr. Timothy Child, "for his able, interesting and instructive address;" but not a word is said about carrying out his suggestions. They do, however, vote to appoint Dr. Oliver W. Holmes, as orator for the next year, thus bringing out their most experienced engineer, to bring to bear his biggest ordnance, and sweep us off forever. And when the year came round, didn't we laugh, that instead of an "infernal machine," to scatter us to the four winds, all we got was a few squibs, and *they* only aimed at the Professor's own little "pedicular" effigy, while a big bombshell was thrown into his own camp, to blow them all sky high.*

For the next act in this interesting drama, we can afford to wait, and, attending to our own business, imitate the example of the good natured husband, who cheerfully submitted to the tirade of his little wife, because it did him no harm, and seemed to do her so much good.

---

* It seems that at an adjourned meeting of the Massachusetts Medical Society, held on the day after the Address was delivered, an exciting discussion occurred on the expediency of publishing sentiments so adapted to undermine the confidence of the public in their mode of practice; and it is understood its publication was advocated only because the effect of suppressing the truth was more to be feared *than the truth itself.*

www.ingramcontent.com/pod-product-compliance
Lightning Source LLC
LaVergne TN
LVHW011138110826
845150LV00008B/2402

* 9 7 8 1 4 1 8 1 9 3 8 5 0 *